THE **Skinny**
5:2 SLOW
FAST DIET COOKER
RECIPE BOOK

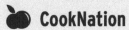

THE SKINNY 5:2 DIET SLOW COOKER RECIPE BOOK

SLOW COOKER RECIPE AND MENU IDEAS UNDER 100, 200, 300 AND 400 CALORIES FOR YOUR 5:2 DIET.

ISBN 978-1482717228

A CIP catalogue record of this book is available from the British Library

DISCLAIMER

Some recipes may contain nuts or traces of nuts. Those suffering from any allergies associated with nuts should avoid any recipes containing nuts or nut based oils.

This information is provided and sold with the knowledge that the publisher and author do not offer any legal or other professional advice.

In the case of a need for any such expertise consult with the appropriate professional.

This book does not contain all information available on the subject, and other sources of recipes are available.

This book has not been created to be specific to any individual's requirements.

Every effort has been made to make this book as accurate as possible. However, there may be typographical and or content errors. Therefore, this book should serve only as a general guide and not as the ultimate source of subject information.

This book contains information that might be dated and is intended only to educate and entertain.

The author and publisher shall have no liability or responsibility to any person or entity regarding any loss or damage incurred, or alleged to have incurred, directly or indirectly, by the information contained in this book.

CONTENTS

SIMPLE LOW CALORIE 5:2 BREAKFAST, SNACK & LUNCH RECIPES

·········· INTRODUCTION ··········

Imagine a diet where you can eat whatever you want for 5 days a week and 'fast' for 2

• •

That's what the 5:2 diet is, and it has revolutionised the way people think about dieting.

By allowing you the freedom to eat normally for MOST of the week and restrict your calorie intake for just TWO days a week (500 calories per day for women and 600 for men) you keep yourself motivated and remove that dreaded feeling of constantly denying yourself the food you really want to eat.

It still takes willpower but is nowhere near as much of a grind when you know that you have tomorrow to look forward to. It's all about freedom. You choose when & what you want to eat, and with the 5:2 Slow Cooker Recipe Book 'diet' can still mean 'delicious'.

Popularised by Dr. Michael J. Mosley, the 5:2 diet plan has been adopted around the world as a way of life, which will change your relationship with dieting and weight loss. What's more, this way of eating is believed to have major health benefits which could alter your health forever.

HOW IT WORKS

The concept of fasting is an ancient one and modern science is uncovering evidence that fasting can be an extremely healthy way to shed extra weight. Research has shown that it can reduce levels of IGF-1 (insulin-like growth factor 1, which leads to accelerated ageing), activate DNA repair genes and reduce blood pressure, cholesterol and glucose levels.

This book has been developed specifically to help you concentrate on the practice of 5:2 Intermittent Fasting, however if you want to find

7

out more about the specific details of the science of the subject we would recommend Dr. Michael J. Mosley's work and, as with all diets, you should consider seeking advice from a health professional before starting.

WHAT THIS BOOK WILL DO FOR YOU

As bestselling Amazon authors of The Skinny Slow Cooker Recipe Book', we noticed lots of 5:2 followers were buying our books, so we decided to put our existing recipes, along with some new ones, into easy-to-use menu planners to support your 5:2 efforts. We know you might still have to cook for the family whilst trying to fast, which is why our healthy slow cooker recipes will help make family mealtimes easy on your fasting days.

For those of you cooking for one, you may also like to try one of CookNations' other best selling titles **'The Skinny 5:2 Fast Diet Meals For One'.**

This book has been designed to get you through your fast days by providing detailed menu plans, recipes and snack ideas to keep you motivated. What makes the 5:2 Diet so good is that it's only a part-time diet. Because you can eat what you want for 5 days a week you will be much more likely to stick with it over time and enjoy the long term health and weight benefits.

TAKING IT WEEK BY WEEK

The 5:2 diet can work for you whatever your lifestyle. Each week you should think carefully about which days are likely to be best suited to your fasting days and then stick with them. You can change your days each week or keep in a regular routine, whichever suits you best.

Of course, reducing your calorie intake for two days will take some getting used to and inevitably there will be hunger pangs to start with, but you'll be amazed at how quickly your body adapts to your new style of eating and, far from gorging the day after your fasting day, you'll find you simply enjoy the luxury of eating normally.

The slow cooker recipes in this book have been designed to fill you up as much as possible during your fasting days. Most recipes serve 4, so if you are cooking only for yourself, freeze into meal-size portions for easy use over the coming weeks. However it's just as likely you will be cooking for others, which is why we've made the recipes family friendly too!

SOME 5:2 TIPS

- Avoid too much exercise on your fasting days. Eating less is likely to make you feel a little weaker, certainly to start with, so don't put pressure on yourself to exercise.
- Avoid alcohol on your fasting days. Not only is alcohol packed with empty calories it could also have a greater effect on you than usual as you haven't eaten as much.
- Don't give up! Even if you find your fasting days tough to start with, stick with it. Remember you can eat what you like tomorrow without having to feel guilty.
- Drink plenty of water throughout the day. Water is the best friend you have on your fasting days. It's good for you, has zero calories, and will fill you up and help stop you feeling hungry.
- When you are eating each meal put your fork down between bites – it will make you eat more slowly and you'll feel fuller on less food.
- Drink a glass of water before and also with your meal. Again this will help you feel fuller.
- Brush your teeth immediately after your meal to discourage yourself from eating more.
- Have clear motivations. Think about what you are trying to achieve and stick with it. Remember you can eat what you want tomorrow.
- If unwanted food cravings do strike, acknowledge them, then distract yourself. Go out for a walk, phone a friend, play with the kids, or paint your nails.
- Whenever hunger hits, try waiting 15 minutes and ride out the cravings. You'll find they usually pass and you can move on with your day.
- Remember - feeling hungry is not a bad thing. We are all so used to acting on the smallest hunger pangs that we forget what it's like to feel genuinely hungry. Feeling hungry for a couple of days a week is not going to harm you. Learn to 'own' your hunger and take control

of how you deal with it.

- If you feel you can't do it by yourself then get some support. Encourage a friend or partner to join you on the 5:2 diet. Having someone to talk things through with can be a real help.
- Get moving. Being active isn't a necessity for the 5:2 Diet to have results but, as with all diets, increased activity will complement your weight loss efforts. Think about what you are doing each day: choose the stairs instead of the lift, walk to the shops instead of driving. Making small changes will not only help you burn calories but will make you feel healthier and more in control of your weight loss.
- Don't beat yourself up! If you have a bad day forget about it, don't feel guilty. Recognise where you went wrong and move on. Tomorrow is a new day and you can start all over again. Fast just two days a week and you'll see results. Guaranteed.

ABOUT OUR SLOW COOKING RECIPES

The recipes in this book are simple and easy to follow, with inexpensive fresh and seasonal ingredients where possible. They are also packed full of flavour and goodness so you can enjoy maximum taste but with minimum calories.

Preparation
These fuss-free recipes are easy and should take no more than 10-15 minutes of preparation - perfect for busy people!
All meat and vegetables should be cut into even-sized pieces unless stated. Although root vegetables can take longer to cook, generally make sure everything is bite-sized and washed before use. Remember that unlike meat, vegetables do not produce their own juices to cook in, so it's important to add the required liquid/stock to each recipe (we've covered this in each list of ingredients). Where our recipes use beans we have used tinned beans for ease. Dried beans are fine too but will require overnight soaking. Meat should be trimmed of visible fat and any skin removed.

Nutrition
All of the recipes in this collection are balanced low-fat family meals which should keep you feeling full and satisfied on your fasting days.

Many have serving suggestions; the calories noted on the recipes are per serving of the recipe ingredients only so bear that in mind.

In any diet it is important to balance your food between proteins, good carbs, dairy, fruit and vegetables.

Protein
Keeps you feeling full and is also essential for building body tissue. Good protein sources come from meat, fish and eggs.

Carbohydrates
Not all carbs are good and generally they are high in calories which makes them difficult to include in a calorie limiting diet. Carbs are a good source of energy for your body as they are converted more easily into glucose (sugar), providing energy. Try to eat 'good carbs' which are high in fibre and nutrients e.g. whole fruits and veg, nuts, seeds, whole grain cereals, beans and legumes.

Dairy
Dairy products provide you with vitamins and minerals. Cheeses can be very high in calories but other products such as low fat Greek yoghurt, crème fraiche and skimmed milk are all good.
Fruit & Veg. Eat your five a day. There is never a better time to fill your 5 a day quota. Not only are fruit and veg very healthy, they also fill up your plate and are ideal snacks when you are feeling hungry.

USING YOUR SLOW COOKER: A FEW THINGS

- All cooking times are a guide. Make sure you get to know your own slow cooker so that you can adjust timings accordingly.
- A spray of one calorie cooking oil in the cooker before adding ingredients will help with cleaning and you can also buy slow cooker liners which make things even easier!
- Be confident with your cooking. Feel free to use substitutes to suit your own taste and don't let a missing herb or spice stop you making a meal - you'll almost always be able to find something to replace it, just be careful it doesn't alter the calorie count.

MEAL PLANNERS

You will soon find out what suits you best on your fasting days by trying out all the different options. It may suit you to skip a meal altogether or you may prefer smaller more regular eats throughout your fasting day. Either way you shouldn't take in more than 500 calories (women) /600 calories (men) per day and this includes drinks.

The menus are based on a 3-week rolling basis. So every option - whether it be leaving out lunch, skipping breakfast or having smaller meals throughout the day - has a 3 week plan of its own.

Not every meal planner is going to work for you, and it may be unrealistic to expect you to use the slow cooker twice a day if you are out at work all day, so feel free to substitute something else for the same calories. Likewise, you may choose to prepare meals in advance so that you can stick with the planners exactly. We have also included non slow cooker snacks, bites and breakfasts to complement the slow cooker recipes and complete the plan for you. That's the beauty of this diet, you can decide how, when and what you eat as long as you stay under 500 calories (women) /600 calories (men) on your fasting days.

We have developed 3 alternative 4-week meal planners to help you.

- OPTION 1:   Skip breakfast, eat lunch & dinner.
- OPTION 2:   Skip lunch, eat breakfast and dinner.
- OPTION 3:   Eat little and often throughout the day.

There is much research and debate about the health benefits and risks of skipping meals, however the beauty of the 5:2 Diet is that the fasting occurs only for 2 days of the week with the remaining 5 reserved for 'normal' eating and recommended daily calorie intakes (1900-2000 for women, 2400-2500 for men). The point being that there is not a prolonged period of starving the body of calories, and eating balanced meals like those included in this book ensures that nutrition is still provided on the fasting days.

ABOUT COOKNATION

CookNation is the leading publisher of innovative and practical recipe books for the modern, health conscious cook.

CookNation titles bring together delicious, easy and practical recipes with their unique approach - easy and delicious, no-nonsense recipes - making cooking for diets and healthy eating fast, simple and fun.

With a range of #1 best-selling titles - from the innovative 'Skinny' calorie-counted series, to the 5:2 Diet Recipes collection - CookNation recipe books prove that 'Diet' can still mean 'Delicious'!

Turn to the end of this book to browse all CookNation's recipe books

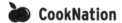 **CookNation**

Skinny

5:2 SLOW
FAST DIET COOKER
LADIES MEAL PLANNERS

....

For fast days where you skip breakfast

....

LADIES FAST DAY MEAL PLANNER WEEK *1*

······ *For fast days where you skip breakfast* ······

500 CALORIES PER FAST DAY

FAST DAY 1		**CALORIES PER SERVING**	**TOTAL DAILY CALORIES**
Drinks Throughout The Day	Tea/Coffee/Low Cal Drinks No more than 50 calories	50	
Lunch	Corn & Potato Chowder (v) (sc)	150	473
Dinner	Best Ever Chicken Curry & Cauliflower Rice (sc)	273	

FAST DAY 2		**CALORIES PER SERVING**	**TOTAL DAILY CALORIES**
Drinks Throughout The Day	Tea/Coffee/Low Cal Drinks No more than 50 calories	50	
Lunch	Bean, Rosemary & Roasted Garlic Dip & Flat Bread (v) (sc)	188	488
Dinner	Tuna & Noodle Cattia (sc)	250	

Notes: Ensure the shop-bought flatbread you have with the homemade bean dip does not exceed 100 calories.

(sc) = slow cooker recipe (v) = vegetarian

RECIPE FINDER

LADIES FAST DAY MEAL PLANNER WEEK 2

······ For fast days where you skip breakfast ······

500 CALORIES PER FAST DAY

FAST DAY 1		CALORIES PER SERVING	TOTAL DAILY CALORIES
Drinks Throughout The Day	Tea/Coffee/Low Cal Drinks No more than 50 calories	50	
Lunch	Slow Spanish Tombet & Plain Tortilla Chips (v) (sc)	169	496
Dinner	Super Simple Chicken Taco Soup & 1 Low Fat Crispbread (sc)	277	

FAST DAY 2		CALORIES PER SERVING	TOTAL DAILY CALORIES
Drinks Throughout The Day	Tea/Coffee/Low Cal Drinks No more than 50 calories	50	
Lunch	Zingy Lime Chicken & 50g Green Salad (sc)	210	500
Dinner	Shepherd-less Pie (v) (sc)	250	

Notes: The shop-bought tortilla chips should be low fat, a portion of 5 chips has been allowed in the calories above.

(sc) = slow cooker recipe (v) = vegetarian

RECIPE FINDER

17

LADIES FAST DAY MEAL PLANNER WEEK 3

...... For fast days where you skip breakfast ......

500 CALORIES PER FAST DAY

FAST DAY 1		CALORIES PER SERVING	TOTAL DAILY CALORIES
Drinks Throughout The Day	Tea/Coffee/Low Cal Drinks No more than 50 calories	50	456
Lunch	Hock Ham & Split Pea Soup (sc)	178	
Dinner	Budapest's Best Beef Goulash (sc)	228	

FAST DAY 2		CALORIES PER SERVING	TOTAL DAILY CALORIES
Drinks Throughout The Day	Tea/Coffee/Low Cal Drinks No more than 50 calories	50	445
Lunch	Asian Hot Soup (v) (sc)	130	
Dinner	Luscious Italian Chicken With 50g Salad & 100g Beansprouts (sc)	265	

(sc) = slow cooker recipe (v) = vegetarian

RECIPE FINDER

Skinny
LADIES MEAL PLANNERS

....

For fast days where you skip lunch

....

NO LUNCH →

LADIES FAST DAY MEAL PLANNER WEEK 1

······ *For fast days where you skip lunch* ······

500 CALORIES PER FAST DAY

FAST DAY 1

		CALORIES PER SERVING	TOTAL DAILY CALORIES
Drinks Throughout The Day	Tea/Coffee/Low Cal Drinks No more than 50 calories	50	
Breakfast	Muesli & 125ml Skimmed Milk (v)	170	496
Dinner	Sweet Asian Chicken & 100g Shirataki Noodles (sc)	276	

FAST DAY 2

		CALORIES PER SERVING	TOTAL DAILY CALORIES
Drinks Throughout The Day	Tea/Coffee/Low Cal Drinks No more than 50 calories	50	
Breakfast	Strawberry & Banana Smoothie & ½ Low Cal Bagel With Low Fat Spread (v)	160	490
Dinner	Sweet & Citrus Salmon & 50g Salad (sc)	280	

Notes: Ensure the shop-bought low calorie bagel does not exceed 100 calories per bagel.

Shirataki noodles are calorie-free noodles which can be bought in most health food shops.

(sc) = slow cooker recipe (v) = vegetarian

RECIPE FINDER

LADIES FAST DAY MEAL PLANNER WEEK 2

⋯⋯ For fast days where you skip lunch ⋯⋯

500 CALORIES PER FAST DAY

FAST DAY 1		CALORIES PER SERVING	TOTAL DAILY CALORIES
Drinks Throughout The Day	Tea/Coffee/Low Cal Drinks No more than 50 calories	50	493
Breakfast	Multigrain Breakfast (v) (sc)	225	
Dinner	Lovely Lemony Garlicky Chicken & 50g Green Salad (sc)	218	

FAST DAY 2		CALORIES PER SERVING	TOTAL DAILY CALORIES
Drinks Throughout The Day	Tea/Coffee/Low Cal Drinks No more than 50 calories	50	488
Breakfast	Mixed Berry Smoothie & 1 Slice Of Wholemeal Toast With Low Fat Spread (v)	180	
Dinner	Sweet & Sour Pineapple Pork & 100g Shirataki Noodles (sc)	258	

Notes: Make sure the wholemeal bread is no more than 70 calories per slice.

Shirataki noodles are calorie-free noodles which can be bought in most health food shops.

(sc) = slow cooker recipe (v) = vegetarian

RECIPE FINDER

LADIES FAST DAY MEAL PLANNER WEEK 3

······ *For fast days where you skip lunch* ······

500 CALORIES PER FAST DAY

FAST DAY 1		CALORIES PER SERVING	TOTAL DAILY CALORIES
Drinks Throughout The Day	Tea/Coffee/Low Cal Drinks No more than 50 calories	50	
Breakfast	Fruit Salad (v)	138	483
Dinner	Lean Green Risotto & 50g Green Salad (v) (sc)	295	

FAST DAY 2		CALORIES PER SERVING	TOTAL DAILY CALORIES
Drinks Throughout The Day	Tea/Coffee/Low Cal Drinks No more than 50 calories	50	
Breakfast	2 Wholegrain Wheat Biscuit Breakfast (e.g. Weetabix) & 125ml Skimmed Milk (v)	198	493
Dinner	Green Thai Fish Curry & Low Fat Rice Cake (sc)	245	

Notes: Make sure the rice cake is no more than 30 calories.

(sc) = slow cooker recipe (v) = vegetarian

RECIPE FINDER

Fruit Salad	page 73
Lean Green Risotto	page 53
Green Thai Fish Curry	page 54

Skinny
LADIES MEAL PLANNERS

....

For fast days where you eat little & often

....

LITTLE & OFTEN ➤

LADIES FAST DAY MEAL PLANNER WEEK *1*

.... *For fast days where you eat little & often* ....

500 CALORIES PER FAST DAY

FAST DAY 1	CALORIES PER SERVING	TOTAL DAILY CALORIES	RECIPE FINDER
Piece Of Fresh Fruit	90		
Nacho, Bean & Onion Dip + Breadsticks (sc)	150		p68
½ Low Fat Bagel & Low Fat Spread	110	**490**	
St. Patrick's Day Soup (sc) (v)	100		p60
Tea/Coffee/Low Cal Drinks No more than 50 calories	50		

FAST DAY 2	CALORIES PER SERVING	TOTAL DAILY CALORIES	RECIPE FINDER
Boiled Egg & 1 Crackerbread	110		
Frozen Banana	90		
Carrot & Celery Salad	97	**488**	p76
Slow Cooked Corn On The Cob (sc) (v)	145		p59
Tea/Coffee/Low Cal Drinks No more than 50 calories	50		

Notes: Breadsticks not to exceed 60 calories.

(sc) = slow cooker recipe (v) = vegetarian

24

LADIES FAST DAY MEAL PLANNER WEEK 2

.... For fast days where you eat little & often ....

500 CALORIES PER FAST DAY

FAST DAY 1	CALORIES PER SERVING	TOTAL DAILY CALORIES	RECIPE FINDER
1 Wedge Water Melon	88		
Corn & Potato Chowder (sc) (v)	150		p61
2 Dutch Crispbakes with 80g Low Fat Cottage Cheese	120	473	
150g Sugar Snap Peas With Sea Salt (sc)	65		p77
Tea/Coffee/Low Cal Drinks No more than 50 calories	50		

FAST DAY 2	CALORIES PER SERVING	TOTAL DAILY CALORIES	RECIPE FINDER
Kiwi & Strawberry Smoothie	100		p84
Tuna With Lemon & Capers	100		p78
Hock Ham & Split Pea Soup (sc)	178	488	p63
12 Plain Pitted Olives	60		
Tea/Coffee/Low Cal Drinks No more than 50 calories	50		

Notes: The shop-bought crispbakes should total no more than 60 calories.

(sc) = slow cooker recipe (v) = vegetarian

LADIES FAST DAY MEAL PLANNER WEEK 3

.... For fast days where you eat little & often ....

500 CALORIES PER FAST DAY

FAST DAY 1	CALORIES PER SERVING	TOTAL DAILY CALORIES	RECIPE FINDER
1 Slice Of Melon With 1 Slice Of Parma Ham	140		
Grilled Chicken & Tomato Snack	100		p75
Handful Of Mixed Berries	80	485	
Slow Spanish Tombet (sc) (v)	115		p55
Tea/Coffee/Low Cal Drinks No more than 50 calories	50		

FAST DAY 2	CALORIES PER SERVING	TOTAL DAILY CALORIES	RECIPE FINDER
150g Blueberries & 1 tbsp Fat Free Greek Yoghurt	140		
Zucchini Soup (sc) (v)	95		p65
100g Low Fat Baked Beans	70	468	
Tomato, Feta & Olive Salad	113		p79
Tea/Coffee/Low Cal Drinks No more than 50 calories	50		

(sc) = slow cooker recipe (v) = vegetarian

Skinny
5:2 SLOW
FAST DIET COOKER
MEN'S MEAL PLANNERS

....

For fast days where you skip breakfast

....

MEN'S FAST DAY MEAL PLANNER WEEK *1*

······ *For fast days where you skip breakfast* ······

600 CALORIES PER FAST DAY

FAST DAY 1		CALORIES PER SERVING	TOTAL DAILY CALORIES
Drinks Throughout The Day	Tea/Coffee/Low Cal Drinks No more than 50 calories	50	**586**
Lunch	Tuna & Pitta Salad	260	
Dinner	Sweet Asian Chicken & 100g Shirataki Noodles (sc)	276	

FAST DAY 2		CALORIES PER SERVING	TOTAL DAILY CALORIES
Drinks Throughout The Day	Tea/Coffee/Low Cal Drinks No more than 50 calories	50	**592**
Lunch	2 Scrambled Eggs On 1 Wholemeal Slice Of Toast	260	
Dinner	Perfect Pulled Pork & 100g Green Salad (sc)	282	

Notes: Shirataki noodles are calorie-free noodles which can be bought in most health food shops

(sc) = slow cooker recipe (V) = vegetarian

RECIPE FINDER

28

MEN'S FAST DAY MEAL PLANNER WEEK 2

...... *For fast days where you skip breakfast* ......

600 CALORIES PER FAST DAY

FAST DAY 1		CALORIES PER SERVING	TOTAL DAILY CALORIES
Drinks Throughout The Day	Tea/Coffee/Low Cal Drinks No more than 50 calories	50	590
Lunch	St.Patrick's Day Soup (sc) (v)	100	
Dinner	Chilli Con Carne (sc)	440	

FAST DAY 2		CALORIES PER SERVING	TOTAL DAILY CALORIES
Drinks Throughout The Day	Tea/Coffee/Low Cal Drinks No more than 50 calories	50	531
Lunch	Zingy Lime Chicken, 100g Green Salad & 1 Slice Avocado	360	
Dinner	Wild Mushroom Stroganoff & 100g Shirataki Noodles (v) (sc)	121	

Notes: Shirataki noodles are calorie-free noodles which can be bought in most health food shops.

(sc) = slow cooker recipe (v) = vegetarian

RECIPE FINDER

St. Patrick's Day Soup — page 60

Chilli Con Carne — page 42

Zingy Lime Chicken — page 56

Wild Mushroom Stroganoff — page 43

MEN'S FAST DAY MEAL PLANNER WEEK 3

...... *For fast days where you skip breakfast* ......

600 CALORIES PER FAST DAY

FAST DAY 1		CALORIES PER SERVING	TOTAL DAILY CALORIES
Drinks Throughout The Day	Tea/Coffee/Low Cal Drinks No more than 50 calories	50	
Lunch	Corn & Potato Chowder (v) (sc)	150	543
Dinner	Italian Meatballs & 100g Green Salad (sc)	343	

FAST DAY 2		CALORIES PER SERVING	TOTAL DAILY CALORIES
Drinks Throughout The Day	Tea/Coffee/Low Cal Drinks No more than 50 calories	50	
Lunch	Nacho, Bean & Onion Dip With Tortilla Chips (v) (sc)	176	599
Dinner	Best Ever Chicken Curry & Cauliflower Rice (sc)	373	

Notes: The shop-bought tortilla chips should be low fat. A portion of 8 chips has been allowed in the calories above.

(sc) = slow cooker recipe (V) = vegetarian

RECIPE FINDER

Skinny
MEN'S MEAL PLANNERS

••

For fast days where you skip lunch

••

NO LUNCH →

MEN'S FAST DAY MEAL PLANNER WEEK *1*

······ For fast days where you skip lunch ······

600 CALORIES PER FAST DAY

FAST DAY 1		CALORIES PER SERVING	TOTAL DAILY CALORIES
Drinks Throughout The Day	Tea/Coffee/Low Cal Drinks No more than 50 calories	50	
Breakfast	Strawberry & Banana Smoothie & Low Cal Bagel With Low Fat Spread (v)	220	538
Dinner	Budapest's Best Beef Goulash, 100g Shirataki Noodles & 100g Green Salad (sc))	268	

FAST DAY 2		CALORIES PER SERVING	TOTAL DAILY CALORIES
Drinks Throughout The Day	Tea/Coffee/Low Cal Drinks No more than 50 calories	50	
Breakfast	Homemade Muesli, 1 tsp Brown Sugar & 125ml Skimmed Milk (v)	204	577
Dinner	Sweet Asian Chicken With 100g Beansprouts & 200g Green Salad (sc)	323	

Notes: Ensure the shop-bought bagel does not exceed 100 calories.

Shirataki noodles are calorie-free noodles which can be bought in most health food shops.

(sc) = slow cooker recipe (v) = vegetarian

RECIPE FINDER

32

MEN'S FAST DAY MEAL PLANNER WEEK 2

······ *For fast days where you skip lunch* ······

600 CALORIES PER FAST DAY

FAST DAY 1		CALORIES PER SERVING	TOTAL DAILY CALORIES
Drinks Throughout The Day	Tea/Coffee/Low Cal Drinks No more than 50 calories	50	597
Breakfast	Fruit Salad & 3 tbsp Fat Free Greek Yoghurt (v)	162	
Dinner	Enchilada El Salvadore, 1 Low Fat Taco Shell & 100g Green Salad (sc)	385	

FAST DAY 2		CALORIES PER SERVING	TOTAL DAILY CALORIES
Drinks Throughout The Day	Tea/Coffee/Low Cal Drinks No more than 50 calories	50	568
Breakfast	3 Wholegrain Wheat Biscuit Breakfast (e.g. Weetabix) & 125ml Skimmed Milk (v)	230	
Dinner	Sweet & Sour Pineapple Pork & Cauliflower Rice (sc)	288	

(sc) = slow cooker recipe (v) = vegetarian

RECIPE FINDER

MEN'S FAST DAY MEAL PLANNER WEEK 3

...... *For fast days where you skip lunch* ......

600 CALORIES PER FAST DAY

FAST DAY 1		CALORIES PER SERVING	TOTAL DAILY CALORIES
Drinks Throughout The Day	Tea/Coffee/Low Cal Drinks No more than 50 calories	50	
Breakfast	Morning Millet & 1 tsp Brown Sugar (v) (sc)	171	576
Dinner	Citrus Salmon, 90g Boiled New Potatoes & 100g Green Salad (sc)	355	

FAST DAY 2		CALORIES PER SERVING	TOTAL DAILY CALORIES
Drinks Throughout The Day	Tea/Coffee/Low Cal Drinks No more than 50 calories	50	
Breakfast	Mixed Berry Smoothie & Frozen Banana (v)	190	580
Dinner	'Hand To Mouth' Tex Mex Tacos With 1 Low Fat Tortilla Wrap, 1 tbsp Low Fat Creme Fraiche, 100g Green Salad & 25g Grated Low Fat Cheese (v) (sc)	340	

(sc) = slow cooker recipe (v) = vegetarian

RECIPE FINDER

Skinny
MEN'S MEAL PLANNERS

....

For fast days where you eat little & often

....

LITTLE & OFTEN

MEN'S FAST DAY MEAL PLANNER WEEK 1

.... For fast days where you eat little & often ....

600 CALORIES PER FAST DAY

FAST DAY 1	CALORIES PER SERVING	TOTAL DAILY CALORIES	RECIPE FINDER
Piece Of Fresh Fruit	90		
Bean, Rosemary & Roasted Garlic Dip + Breadsticks (sc)	150		p67
½ Low Fat Bagel & Low Fat Spread	110	595	
Zucchini Soup (sc) (v)	95		p65
1 tbsp Sunflower Seeds	90		
Tea/Coffee/Low Cal Drinks No more than 50 calories	50		

FAST DAY 2	CALORIES PER SERVING	TOTAL DAILY CALORIES	RECIPE FINDER
Boiled Egg & 1 Slice Of Wholemeal Toast	160		
Frozen Banana @ Babybel Light Cheese Portion	133		
Carrot & Celery Salad	97	585	p76
Slow Cooked Corn On The Cob (sc) (v)	150		p59
Tea/Coffee/Low Cal Drinks No more than 50 calories	50		

Notes: Breadsticks not to exceed 60 calories. Ensure shop-bought bagel does not exceed 100 calories. Shop-bought bread should not exceed 60 calories per slice.

(sc) = slow cooker recipe (v) = vegetarian

MEN'S FAST DAY MEAL PLANNER WEEK 2

.... For fast days where you eat little & often ....

600 CALORIES PER FAST DAY

FAST DAY 1	CALORIES PER SERVING	TOTAL DAILY CALORIES	RECIPE FINDER
3 tbsp Homemade Salsa & 2 Carrots Cut Into Batons	100		p81
Barley & Chestnut Mushroom Soup (sc) (v)	175		p66
200g Shirataki Noodles With 1 tbsp Soy Sauce & Pinch Of Chilli Flakes	70	560	
150g Sugar Snap Peas With Sea Salt (sc)	65		p77
Small Apple Cut In Slices With 2 tsp Low Fat Peanut Butter	100		
Tea/Coffee/Low Cal Drinks No more than 50 calories	50		

FAST DAY 2	CALORIES PER SERVING	TOTAL DAILY CALORIES	RECIPE FINDER
1 Hard Boiled Egg	100		
25g Pistachios	127		
Wild Mushroom Stroganoff (v) (sc)	101	578	p43
½ cup/120ml Fat Free Greek Yogurt With 1tsp Runny Honey	90		
150g Strawberries With 1tsp Brown Sugar	110		
Tea/Coffee/Low Cal Drinks No more than 50 calories	50		

Notes: Shirataki noodles are calorie-free noodles which can be bought in most health food shops.

(sc) = slow cooker recipe (v) = vegetarian

MEN'S FAST DAY MEAL PLANNER WEEK 3

.... For fast days where you eat little & often ....

600 CALORIES PER FAST DAY

FAST DAY 1	CALORIES PER SERVING	TOTAL DAILY CALORIES	RECIPE FINDER
1 Wedge Of Water Melon	88		
Corn & Potato Chowder (sc) (v)	150		p61
2 Dutch Crispbakes With 80g Low Fat Cottage Cheese	120	598	
Kiwi & Strawberry Smoothie	100		p84
Muller Light Yogurt	90		
Tea/Coffee/Low Cal Drinks No more than 50 calories	50		

FAST DAY 2	CALORIES PER SERVING	TOTAL DAILY CALORIES	RECIPE FINDER
20g Cashew Nuts	100		
Tuna With Lemon & Capers	101		p78
Hock Ham & Split Pea Soup (sc)	178	599	p63
18 Pitted Olives	90		
Dozen Whole Almonds	80		
Tea/Coffee/Low Cal Drinks No more than 50 calories	50		

Notes: The shop-bought crispbakes should total no more than 60 calories.

(sc) = slow cooker recipe (v) = vegetarian

Skinny

5:2 SLOW

FAST DIET COOKER

RECIPES

SERVES 6

PERFECT PULLED PORK

calories per
serving

Ingredients

- 800g/1 ¾lb lean pork butt
  (shoulder)
- 1 onion, chopped
- 60ml/¼ cup BBQ sauce or ketchup
- 250ml/1 cup beef stock/broth
- 1 packet BBQ dry rub

Or make your own:
- 1 tbsp each of garlic powder,
  brown sugar, onion powder,
- celery salt, paprika
- 1 tsp each mild chilli powder &
  cumin

Method

1 Combine all the spices together and cover the pork in the dry rub.

2 Add the stock, onion & BBQ sauce and place the pork on top. Leave to cook on high for 4-6 hours with the lid tightly closed. Ideally you should turn the pork half way through cooking but if you can't don't worry too much.

3 Once the pork is super-tender remove it from the slow cooker. Leave to rest for as long as you can resist and then use your hands or two forks to pull the pork apart.

4 Once it's all shredded place in a bowl and remove the cooking liquid from the slow cooker.

5 Pour the liquid onto the pork to make beautiful juicy meat.

Family Serving Suggestion (Not 5:2 Followers): Salad, rolls and barbecue sauce.

CHEFS NOTE
Pulled pork is an absolute classic. It's a chance to use just about everything in your spice rack to create a killer dry rub and it always packs an irresistible punchy and more-ish taste.

SWEET ASIAN CHICKEN

256 calories per serving

.... *Ingredients* ....

- 500g/1lb 2oz skinless chicken breasts
- 2 garlic cloves, crushed
- 1 onion, chopped
- 60ml/¼ cup honey
- 2 tbsp tomato puree/paste
- 4 tbsp light soy sauce
- 2 carrots, cut into batons

- Pinch crushed chilli
- 120ml/½ cup fresh orange juice
- 2 tsp sunflower oil
- 1 tsp cornstarch/cornflour dissolved in a little water to form a paste

.... *Method* ....

1 Combine all the ingredients in a bowl and add to the slow cooker.

2 Cook on low for 5-6 hours or on high 3-4 hours with the lid tightly shut.

3 When the chicken is cooked through and tender, season and serve.

Family Serving Suggestion (Not 5:2 Followers): Fine egg noodles, rice & chopped spring onions.

CHEFS NOTE

The honey, soy and orange juice in this dish make it a hit with the kids and adds a little eastern flavour to evening meal times.

CHILLI CON CARNE

Ingredients

- 550g/1¼lb lean minced beef
- 400g/14oz tinned chopped tomatoes
- 200g/7oz tinned kidney beans, drained
- 1 large onion, chopped
- 250ml/1 cup beef stock
- 500ml/2 cups tomato passata/ sauce
- 1 tsp each of brown sugar, oregano, cumin, chilli powder, paprika & garlic
- ½ tsp salt
- Low cal cooking oil spray

Method

1 Use a little low cal spray to brown the mince and onions in a frying pan.

2 Add all the ingredients into the slow cooker and combine well.

3 Leave to cook on low for 5-6 hours or high 3-4 hours with the lid tightly closed or until the meat is tender and cooked through.

Family Serving Suggestion (Not 5:2 Followers): Rice, tortilla chips and a dollop of fat free Greek yoghurt.

CHEFS NOTE

The Spanish name simply means 'chilli with meat' and this dish has been a Tex-Mex classic since before the days of the American frontier settlers. Slow cooking the minced beef really allows the flavour to develop.

WILD MUSHROOM STROGANOFF

101
calories per serving

············· *Ingredients* ···············

- 675g/1½lb wild mixed mushrooms sliced
- 2 large onions, sliced
- 4 garlic cloves, crushed
- 2 teaspoons smoked paprika
- 250ml/1 cup vegetable stock

- 400g/14oz tinned low fat condensed mushroom soup
- ½ tsp butter
- Bunch flat chopped leaf parsley (reserve a little for garnish)

··············· *Method* ···················

1 Add all the ingredients into the slow cooker.

2 Close the lid tightly and leave to cook on high for 2-3 hours or low 4-5 hours.

3 Check the seasoning and serve.

Family Serving Suggestion (Not 5:2 Followers):
Pasta or rice.

CHEFS NOTE
The more exciting the mushrooms the better this dish is going to taste. Use whatever you can get your hands on, a combination of Portobello, Shitake, Morel, Oyster and Enoki would be fantastic, but don't be put off if you can only get regular varieties.

ITALIAN MEATBALLS

323
calories per
serving

Ingredients

- 650g/1lb 7oz lean minced/ground beef
- 1 slice of bread whizzed into breadcrumbs
- 1 onion, finely chopped
- Handful of fresh flat leaf parsley chopped
- 1 large egg

- 1 clove garlic, crushed
- 1 tsp salt
- 800g/1¾lb tinned chopped tomatoes
- 2 tbsp tomato puree/paste
- 250ml/1 cup beef stock
- 1 tsp each of dried basil, oregano & thyme

Method

1 Combine together the beef, breadcrumbs, onion, egg, garlic and half a teaspoon of salt. (You can do it with your hands or for super speed put it all into a food mixer).

2 Once the ingredients are properly mixed together use your hands to shape into about 20-24 meat balls.

3 Add all the ingredients to the slow cooker and combine well.

4 Leave to cook with the lid tightly on for 5-6 hours or 3-4 hours on high.

5 Ensure the beef is well cooked.

CHEFS NOTE
Meatballs are easy to make and never a disappointment to eat. The simple sauce accompanying the meat here is lovely as it is, but a dash of Worcestershire sauce or a teaspoon of marmite will give it additional depth.

Family Serving Suggestion (Not 5:2 Followers):
Spaghetti & Parmesan Cheese.

BUDAPEST'S BEST BEEF GOULASH

228
calories per serving

.... *Ingredients* ....

- 800g/1¾lb lean stewing steak, cubed (trim off any fat you can)
- 1 red pepper, deseeded & sliced
- 3 garlic cloves, crushed
- 250ml/1 cup beef stock
- 250ml/1 cup red wine
- 400g/14oz tinned chopped tomatoes

- 1 tbsp tomato puree/paste
- 1 tsp paprika
- 1 tbsp plain/all purpose flour
- 1 large onion, chopped
- Salt & pepper to taste
- Low cal cooking oil spray

.... *Method* ....

1 Season the beef with salt and pepper and quickly brown in a smoking hot pan with a little low cal spray.

2 Remove from pan and dust with flour (the easiest way is to put the beef and flour into a plastic bag and give it a good shake).

3 Add all the ingredients to the slow cooker and combine well. Leave to cook on Low with the lid tightly on for 5-6 hours.

4 Ensure the beef is tender and cooked through and, if you want to thicken it up a little, leave to cook for a further 45 mins with the lid off.

Family Serving Suggestion (Not 5:2 Followers): Salad, sour cream and tagliatelle pasta.

CHEFS NOTE
Goulash is a European dish which suits the slow cooker beautifully. After hours of gentle cooking this 'tougher' meat becomes a tender cut which melts in the mouth. meatbecomes a tender cut which melts in the mouth.

ENCHILADA EL SALVADOR

324
calories per serving

Ingredients

- 450g/1lb lean minced beef/ground beef
- 1 onion chopped
- 1 green pepper, deseeded & chopped
- 200g/7oz tinned black beans, drained
- 400g/14oz tinned chopped tomatoes
- 250ml/1 cup beef stock
- Chilli to taste!
- 4 tsp your favourite packet taco seasoning

Or make your own:
- 2 tsp mild chilli powder
- 1½tsp ground cumin
- ½ tsp paprika
- ¼ tsp each of onion powder, garlic powder, dried oregano & crushed chilli flakes,
- 1 tsp each of sea salt & black pepper

Method

1 Add all the ingredients to the slow cooker and combine well.

2 Leave to cook with the lid tightly on for 5-6 hours or 3-4 hours on high.

3 Ensure the beef is well cooked, if you want to thicken up a little leave to cook for a further 45 mins with the lid off.

Family Serving Suggestion (Not 5:2 Followers):
Flour tortillas, shredded salad, grated cheese and sour cream.

CHEFS NOTE
Inspired by the flavours of Tex Mex this dish is great fun to eat as a family with everyone helping themselves across the table, making their own perfect enchilada!

SWEET & SOUR PINEAPPLE PORK

238 calories per serving

Ingredients

- 2lb or 900g tenderloin pork fillet, cubed
- 1 tbsp plain/all purpose flour
- 200g/7oz tinned pineapple chunks (reserve the juice)
- 1 onion chopped
- 1 green pepper, deseeded & chopped

- 2 carrots, cut into batons
- 1 tbsp brown sugar
- ½ tsp salt
- 2 tbsp lime juice
- 1 tbsp light soy sauce
- 120ml/½ cup chicken stock
- Low cal cooking oil spray

Method

1 Brown the pork in a frying pan with a little low cal spray. Remove from the pan and dust with flour.

2 Put all the other ingredients, except the pineapple chunks, into the slow cooker (including the pineapple juice).

3 Combine everything and leave to cook on low for 6-8 hours with the lid tightly closed.

4 Check the pork is tender, add the pineapple chunks and cook for a further 30 min.

Family Serving Suggestion (Not 5:2 Followers): Boiled rice and prawn crackers.

CHEFS NOTE

Sweet and Sour is one of the most loved Chinese meals in the world. This is not supposed to be an authentic copy, just take it as a super-simple replica which should satisfy your Eastern cravings!

SWEET & CITRUS SALMON

270
calories per serving

Ingredients

- 4 boneless salmon fillets, each weighing 150g/5oz
- 1 onion, chopped
- 60ml/¼ cup light soy sauce
- 4 tbsp lime juice
- 2 garlic cloves, crushed
- 200g/7oz green beans
- 1 tbsp honey
- Low cal cooking oil spray

Method

1 Sauté the onion and garlic for a few minutes in a little low cal spray.

2 Brush the salmon fillets with the honey. Remove from the pan and carefully combine all the ingredients in the slow cooker.

3 Cook on low for 1½ hours with the lid tightly on. Check the salmon is properly cooked by flaking it a little with a fork.

4 Season and serve.

CHEFS NOTE

Salmon can be relatively expensive so feel free to substitute for tilapia or basa, or talk to your fishmonger for recommendations.

Family Serving Suggestion (Not 5:2 Followers):
Boiled salad potatoes or rice..

BEST EVER CHICKEN CURRY

223
calories per
serving

Ingredients

- 500g/1lb 2oz skinless chicken breasts, cubed
- 1 onion, chopped
- 1 tbsp tomato puree/paste
- 3 cloves garlic crushed
- 1 tsp low-fat butter spread
- 1 tbsp freshly grated ginger (or 1 tsp of ginger powder)

- 1 tsp each garam masala, ground cumin & turmeric
- 25ml/1 cup tomato passata/ sauce
- ½ tsp chilli powder
- 4 tbsp fat free Greek yoghurt
- Pinch salt

Method

1 Combine all the ingredients, except the yoghurt, in the slow cooker.

2 Cook on low for 5-6 hours, or on high 3-4 hours with the lid tightly shut.

3 Ensure the chicken is cooked through and tender, turn off the heat and stir in the yoghurt.

Family Serving Suggestion (Not 5:2 Followers):
Salad, rolls and barbecue sauce.

CHEFS NOTE

Curry has never been more popular across the world The mix of spices below is preferable but it's fine to substitute with curry powder if you are in a rush or struggling with store cupboard ingredients.

49

HAND TO MOUTH TEX MEX TACOS

150
calories per
serving

Ingredients

- 200g/14oz tinned black beans, drained & rinsed
- 400g/14oz tinned chopped tomatoes
- 1 courgette/zucchini, chopped
- 1 green pepper, deseeded & chopped

- 1 tsp paprika
- ½ tsp each chilli powder & garlic powder
- 1 tsp each oregano, thyme, cumin and onion powder
- 50g/2oz rice
- 120ml/½ cup vegetable stock

Method

1 Combine all the ingredients into the slow cooker and cook on low for 6-8 hours with the lid tightly closed or on high 4-6 hours.

Family Serving Suggestion (Not 5:2 Followers): Taco shells, avocado, lettuce, salsa, cheese, onions and sour cream.

2 Check the rice is tender and add more water during cooking if necessary.

3 If you want to thicken the taco take the lid off and continue to cook on high for 45 mins or until the consistency is right for you.

CHEFS NOTE
Tacos are traditionally eaten with hands not utensils and this tasty version should be no different. Enjoy with friends who don't mind messy eaters!

TUNA & NOODLE CATTIA

250 calories per serving

.... *Ingredients* ....

- 350g/12oz fresh egg noodles
- 1 onion, chopped
- 400g/14oz tin fat-free condensed mushroom soup
- 400g/14oz tinned tuna
- 100g/3½oz frozen peas
- 1 tsp garlic powder
- Pinch Salt
- Pinch of crushed chilli flakes

.... *Method* ....

1 Quickly cook the pasta or noodles in salted boiling water for a minute or two.

2 Save 3 tbsp of the drained water and then combine it, along with all the ingredients in the slow cooker and cook on low for 1½ hours.

Family Serving Suggestion (Not 5:2 Followers): Sliced red onion and tomato salad with Parmesan cheese.

CHEFS NOTE
An absolute classic American slow cooker recipe. This version takes it back to basics using the simplest store cupboard ingredients. e.

SERVES 4

LUSCIOUS ITALIAN CHICKEN

235 calories per serving

Ingredients

- 400g/14oz skinless chicken breasts
- 400g/14oz tinned low fat condensed chicken or mushroom soup
- 100g/3½ oz sliced mushrooms
- 1 onion, chopped
- Pinch salt
- Clove garlic crushed
- 2 tbsp low fat cream cheese
- Dried rub mix of:
- 1 tsp each oregano, rosemary & thyme

Method

1 Rub chicken breasts with the dried herbs mix and combine all the ingredients into the slow cooker.

2 Cook on low for 5-6 hours or on high 3-4 hours with the lid tightly shut.

3 Ensure the chicken is cooked through and tender. Add a little chicken stock during cooking if needed.

Family Serving Suggestion (Not 5:2 Followers): Vegetbales, spaghetti or rice.

CHEFS NOTE
With a lovely creamy consistency this Italian inspired dish makes the most of that wonderful 'cheat' ingredient 'condensed soup'!

LEAN GREEN RISOTTO

285 calories per serving

Ingredients

- 1 tbsp olive oil
- Knob of butter
- 1 large onion, chopped
- 2 cloves of garlic, chopped
- 225g/8oz risotto rice
- 1lt/4cups vegetable stock
- 1 tsp green pesto
- 125g/4oz sliced green beans, chopped
- 125g/4oz frozen peas
- 125g/4oz spinach, chopped

Method

1 Saute the onion in the oil and butter for a few minutes.

2 Add the risotto to the pan and make sure each grain is coated well with the oil and butter.

3 Transfer to the slow cooker and combine all the ingredients. Leave to cook on High for 2-3 hours with the lid tightly shut, the risotto may need a little water during cooking so check if you can every half hour or so.

Family Serving Suggestion (Not 5:2 Followers): Basil & rocket salad with Parmesan shavings.

CHEFS NOTE
Usually served as a first course in Italy, this veggie pesto version makes a beautiful main course.

GREEN THAI FISH CURRY

215
calories per serving

Ingredients

- 500g/1 lb 2oz boneless, white fish fillets (go for whatever is on sale) haddock, cod, pollock, cobbler... all meaty white fish will work well
- 2 onions, chopped
- 1 tsp freshly grated ginger or ½ tsp ground ginger
- 3 cloves garlic, crushed

- 1 whole red chilli
- 2 large handfuls watercress
- 2 tbsp Thai green curry paste
- 250ml/1 cup low fat coconut milk
- 1 tsp sunflower oil
- Pinch salt

Method

1 Sauté the onions & green beans with the ginger and garlic over a low heat in the sunflower oil.

2 Season the fish fillets with salt and pepper and carefully combine all the ingredients (except the watercress) in the slow cooker.

3 Cover and cook on low for 1½ hours. This timing should mean the fish is not overcooked and the green beans still have some bite to them.

4 Check the fish is properly cooked through by flaking it a little with a fork and gently add the watercress before serving.

Family Serving Suggestion (Not 5:2 Followers):
Rice or noodles.

CHEFS NOTE

Compared to meat, fish cooks more quickly in the slow cooker and as such fish recipes can be really handy if you haven't got too much cooking time. This recipe is a fantastic and really easy Thai curry which, is simple to prepare and doesn't take long at all in the slow cooker.

SLOW SPANISH TOMBET

115 calories per serving

Ingredients

- 2 aubergines/eggplant, cubed
- 2 courgettes/zucchini, cut into strips
- 4 fresh tomatoes, cubed
- 2 red peppers, deseeded & sliced
- 4 tbsp tomato puree/paste
- 2 red onions, 1 chopped, 1 sliced
- 1 tsp each of dried marjoram, basil & thyme
- ½ tsp paprika
- 1 tsp capers
- Handful pitted black olives
- 3 garlic cloves, crushed
- 1 tsp salt
- 1 tsp sugar
- 1 tbsp olive oil
- 120ml/½ cup vegetable stock
- Fresh basil to garnish

Method

1 Combine all ingredients in the slow cooker, cover and leave to cook on low for 4-5 hours/high for 2-3 hours or until the vegetables are tender.

2 If you want to thicken the sauce take the lid off and continue to cook on high for 45 mins or until the consistency is right for you.

Family Serving Suggestion (Not 5:2 Followers): Spanish toast (rough cut farmhouse bread toasted and rubbed with garlic, salt & olive oil).

CHEFS NOTE
Tombet is the Spanish version of the French classic ratatouille.

ZINGY LIME CHICKEN

200
calories per serving

Ingredients

- 500g/1lb 2oz chicken breasts
- 2 tbsp lime juice
- Bunch fresh coriander, chopped
- 1 green chilli, deseeded & finely chopped
- 200g/7oz salsa

Or make your own salsa:

- Add 1 onion chopped, 1 clove garlic crushed, 1 green chilli chopped to 2 x regular cans (14 oz/400 g) chopped tomatoes + sea salt to taste

- 4 tsp your favourite packet taco seasoning

Or make your own taco seasoning:

- 2 tsp mild chilli powder, 1 ½ tsp ground cumin, ½ tsp paprika, ¼ tsp each of onion powder, garlic powder, dried oregano & crushed chilli flakes + 1 tsp each of sea salt & black pepper

Method

1 Put everything together in the slow cooker making sure the chicken is covered with the rest of the ingredients.

2 With the lid tightly shut leave to cook for 4-5 hours on high or 6-8 hours on the low setting.

3 Ensure the chicken is cooked through and tender then shred it a little with two forks, season and serve.

Family Serving Suggestion (Not 5:2 Followers):
Green salad, rice or quesadillas (flour tortillas).

CHEFS NOTE
Packed with protein, chicken breasts are a fantastic low-fat meat to use in the slow cooker. The citrus lightness of this recipe is perfect for all seasons.

SERVES 4

SHEPHERD-LESS PIE

240
calories per serving

Ingredients

- 1 tbsp olive oil
- 1 onions, chopped
- 2 carrots, diced
- 2 stalks celery, chopped
- 1 garlic clove, crushed chopped
- 75g/3oz mushrooms, sliced
- 1 bay leaf
- 1 tsp dried thyme
- 75g/3oz dried green lentils (soaked

- overnight)
- splash red wine if you have it
- 1 tbsp Worcestershire sauce/ A1 steak sauce
- 250ml/1 cup vegetable stock
- 2 tbsp tomato purée/paste
- 600g/1lb 5oz mashed potato to top the pie

Method

1 Gently sauté the onions, celery, carrots and garlic in the herbs for a few minutes.

2 Remove to the slow cooker and combine well with all the other ingredients (except the mashed potato) and leave to cook on low for 4-5 hours with the lid tightly closed, or on high for 2-3 hours. If you want to thicken the sauce take the lid off and continue to cook on high for 45 mins or until the consistency is right for you.

3 Remove from the slow cooker and place in a oven proof dish.

4 Top with the mashed potato and brown under the grill for a few minutes.

Family Serving Suggestion (Not 5:2 Followers):
Peas and spring greens dressed with garlic oil.

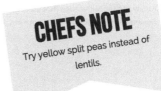
CHEFS NOTE
Try yellow split peas instead of lentils.

LOVELY LEMONY GARLICKY CHICKEN

208
calories per
serving

Ingredients

- 500g/1lb 2oz skinless chicken breasts
- 3 garlic cloves, crushed
- 2 whole lemons sliced
- 1 onion, chopped
- 1 tsp honey

- 1 tsp cornstarch/cornflour dissolved in a little water to form a paste
- 500ml/2 cups chicken stock
- Salt & pepper to taste
- Bunch fresh Basil, chopped

Method

1 Combine all the ingredients in your slow cooker and leave to cook on low for 5-6 hours or on high 3-4 hours with the lid tightly shut.

2 Ensure the chicken is cooked through and tender.

Family Serving Suggestion (Not 5:2 Followers):
Steamed vegetables and new potatoes.

CHEFS NOTE
This is a really simple dish which benefits from using fresh lemons and fresh basil ideally.

SLOW COOKED CORN ON THE COB

145 calories per serving

········· *Ingredients* ············

- 1 medium ear of fresh sweetcorn
- 1 clove garlic, crushed
- 1 tsp low fat spread
- Salt & pepper to taste

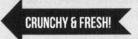
CRUNCHY & FRESH!

········· *Method* ············

1 Mix the low fat spread and garlic in a bowl, coat the sweetcorn with this mix and wrap in foil.

2 Place in the slow cooker and leave to cook on high with the lid tightly shut for 2 hours or until tender.

Family Serving Suggestion (Not 5:2 Followers):
Salad, rolls and barbecue sauce.

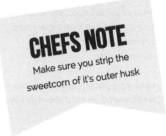
CHEFS NOTE
Make sure you strip the sweetcorn of it's outer husk

ST. PATRICK'S DAY SOUP

100
calories per
serving

Ingredients

- 225g/8oz potatoes, chopped
- 1 large onion, chopped
- 3 leeks, chopped
- Salt & pepper to taste

- 250ml/1 cup semi skimmed/
  half fat milk
- 750ml/3 cups vegetable stock

Method

1 Combine all the ingredients together in the slow cooker and leave to cook on low for 3-4hours with the lid tightly shut.

2 Make sure the potatoes are tender, season to taste and then either blend as a smooth soup or eat it rough, ready and rustic.

Family Serving Suggestion (Not 5:2 Followers):
Crusty bread, sour cream and chopped parsley.

CHEFS NOTE
It's often said that everyone is Irish on St. Patrick's day and here's a chance to get a real taste of Ireland every day with this lovely potato soup.

CORN & POTATO CHOWDER

150 calories per serving

Ingredients

- 1 onion, chopped
- 400g/14oz sweetcorn
- 400g/14oz tinned creamed sweetcorn
- 2 garlic cloves, crushed
- 750ml/3 cups vegetable stock
- 250g/9oz potatoes, diced
- 1 tsp low fat butter spread
- 250ml/1 cup semi skimmed/ half fat milk
- 1 tsp salt

Method

1 Sauté the onion and garlic in a little low cal cooking spray.

2 Place all the ingredients in the slow cooker and cook on low for 3-4 hours with the lid tightly shut.

3 Ensure the potatoes are tender , mash a little with a fork to create the right consistency.

4 Season and serve.

Family Serving Suggestion (Not 5:2 Followers): Saltine or cream crackers.

CHEFS NOTE

Although usually associated with seafood, chowder is a lovely thick soup which works just as well with vegetables alone. You could easily add some smoked haddock to this recipe if you like.

SUPER SIMPLE CHICKEN TACO SOUP

247 calories per serving

Ingredients

- 125g/4oz skinless chicken breast
- 200g/7oz sweetcorn
- 200g/7oz tinned kidney beans
- 400g/14oz tinned chopped tomatoes
- 2 cloves garlic, crushed
- 1lt/4 cups warm water
- 1 chilli chopped or a pinch of dried crushed chilli flakes (add as much as you like)

- 4 tsp your favourite packet taco seasoning

Or make your own taco seasoning:
- 2 tsp mild chilli powder, 1 ½ tsp ground cumin, ½ tsp paprika, ¼ tsp each of onion powder, garlic powder, dried oregano & crushed chilli flakes + 1 tsp each of sea salt & black pepper
-

Method

1 Season the chicken and place at the bottom of the slow cooker. Add all the other ingredients and leave to cook for 2 hours on high or 3 hours on low with the lid tightly shut.

2 Ensure the chicken is cooked through and tender, then shred it a little with 2 forks through the soup.

3 If you want to thicken the soup, take the lid off and cook on high for a further 45minutes or until you get the consistency you want.

Family Serving Suggestion (Not 5:2 Followers):
Tortilla chips, crusty bread or over rice.

CHEFS NOTE
No one knows when Taco turned into soup, but whenever it was it's a firm favourite which is worth celebrating in the slow cooker.

HOCK HAM & SPLIT PEA SOUP

178
calories per serving

Ingredients

- 2 ham knuckles (smoked are best)
- 3 carrots, chopped
- 2 celery stalks, chopped
- 1 onion, chopped

- 3 garlic cloves, crushed
- 200g/7oz green or yellow split peas (soaked overnight)
- 1lt/4 cups chicken stock

Method

1 Combine all the ingredients into the slow cooker and cook on low for 4-5 hours or high for 2-3 hours with the lid tightly shut.

2 When the soup is cooked take out the hocks and strip them of any meat, if they are fully cooked the meat should fall away easily.

3 Get rid of any fat and stir the shredded ham back into the soup.

4 If you want to alter the texture you can thicken it up by mashing the split peas a little before putting the ham meat back in.

CHEFS NOTE

Ham hocks are a bargain ingredient that can add a real depth to a dish. You could substitute ham hocks for a meaty ham bone if you had one left after a family gathering.

ASIAN HOT SOUP

130
calories per
serving

Ingredients

- 50g/2oz shiitake mushrooms
- 50g/2oz cloud ear fungus (if you can get them or closed cap if you can't)
- 200g/7oz tinned bamboo shoots, drained
- 3 cloves garlic, crushed
- 1 tsp sesame oil
- 1 tsp chilli paste (or dried crushed chillies to taste)
- 2 tbsp rice wine vinegar or wine vinegar
- 225g/8oz frozen peas
- 2 tbsp soy sauce
- 1 tsp sesame oil
- 275g/10oz tofu, cubed
- 1 tbsp freshly grated ginger
- 750ml/3 cups vegetable stock

Method

1 Combine all the ingredients in your slow cooker and leave to cook of low 6-8 hours with the lid tightly shut or high for 3-6 hours.

2 Season and serve.Pour the liquid onto the pork to make beautiful juicy meat.

CHEFS NOTE
This is a lovely version of Chinese Hot & Sour soup, load up on fresh immune boosting ginger if you can handle it.

ZUCCHINI SOUP

95 calories per serving

Ingredients

- 50g/2oz potato, cubed
- 500ml/2 cups vegetable stock
- 1 small head broccoli, chopped
- ½ cauliflower, chopped
- 1 tsp each cumin and paprika
- Salt to taste

- 1 tsp olive oil
- 1 onion
- 2 garlic cloves, crushed
- 2 courgettes/zucchini, chopped

Method

1 Gently sauté the onion and courgettes in the oil for a couple of minutes.

2 Add all the ingredients into the slow cooker and leave to cook on low for 6-8 hours or high for 3-4 hours with the lid tightly shut.

3 Blend soup to required consistency, season and serve.

Family Serving Suggestion (Not 5:2 Followers):
Grated Parmesan or crumbled stilton cheese.

CHEFS NOTE
Add a little milk or fat free Greek yoghurt for a creamy texture

BARLEY & CHESTNUT MUSHROOM SOUP

175 calories per serving

Ingredients

- 1 large onion, chopped
- 1 tsp olive oil
- 1 carrot, chopped
- 1 celery stalk, chopped
- 200g/7oz mushrooms finely chopped
- 400g/14oz tinned chopped tomatoes

- 200g/7oz frozen sweetcorn
- 75g/3oz pearl barley
- 1 tsp each of basil, oregano, thyme
- Salt & pepper to taste
- 3 cloves garlic, crushed
- 1lt/4 cups vegetable stock

Method

1 Gently sauté the onions, carrot, mushrooms and celery in a frying pan with the oil for a few minutes until softened.

2 Combine all the ingredients into the slow cooker and cook on low for 5-6 hours with the lid tightly closed or on high 4-6 hours.

3 Season and serve.

CHEFS NOTE
This is a really tasty and filling soup. The mushrooms should be finely chopped to give the soup some body.

BEAN, ROSEMARY AND ROASTED GARLIC DIP

88 calories per serving

Ingredients

- 6 garlic cloves, chopped
- 50g/2oz Parmesan cheese, grated
- 1 bunch chopped fresh rosemary
- 1 tbsp extra virgin olive oil
- 300g/11oz tin borlotti beans, drained
- 75g/3oz low fat cream cheese

- Handful chopped black olives
- 1 tbsp white wine vinegar
- 250ml/1 cup water
- 1 tbsp lemon juice
- Salt to taste

Method

1 Quickly pulse all the ingredients (except the lemon juice) in a food processor.

2 Empty the blitzed mixture into the slow cooker and leave to cook on low for 1-2 hours.

3 If the mixture it too thick add a little more water. If it's not thick enough continue to cook with the lid off until you get the required consistency.

4 After cooking allow to cool and stir in the lemon juice.

Family Serving Suggestion (Not 5:2 Followers):
Flat bread, cucmber & carrot batons.

CHEFS NOTE
Kalamata olives are particularly good in this recipe.

67

NACHO BEAN & ONION DIP

90 calories per serving

Ingredients

- 800g/1 ¾lb tinned low fat refried beans
- 1 green chilli, deseeded & finely chopped
- 1 large onion chopped
- 250ml/1 cup water
- 100g/3½oz low fat mozzarella cheese chopped
- 1 packet of your favourite taco seasoning mix

Or make your own taco seasoning:
- 2 tsp mild chilli powder, 1 ½ tsp ground cumin, ½ tsp paprika, ¼ tsp each of onion powder, garlic powder, dried oregano & crushed chilli flakes, 1 tsp each of sea salt & black pepper
- Salt to taste
- 1 tbsp lemon juice

Method

1 Place all the ingredients, except the lemon juice, into the slow cooker and combine well. Leave to cook on low for 1-2 hours.

2 If the mixture is too thick add a little more water. If it's not thick enough continue to cook with the lid off until you get the required consistency.

3 Stir in the lemon juice before serving.

Family Serving Suggestion (Not 5:2 Followers): Tortilla chips or breadsticks.

MULTI GRAIN BREAKFAST

225
calories per serving

Ingredients

- 25g/1oz rolled oats
- 75g /3oz bulgur wheat
- 50g/2oz brown rice
- 25g/1oz pearl barley
- 50g/2oz quinoa
- 150g/5oz chopped apple (no need to peel)

- 75g/3oz raisins
- 1 tsp ground cinnamon
- 2 tsp vanilla extract
- 750ml/3 cups water
- Sprinkle of nutmeg

Method

1 Combine all the ingredients (except the nutmeg) in the slow cooker and leave to cook overnight on low for 6 to 8 hours with the lid tightly shut.

2 Add more water if needed and stir well. Sprinkle with nutmeg after cooking.

Family Serving Suggestion (Not 5:2 Followers): Add vanilla soymilk and organic maple syrup to your taste.

CHEFS NOTE
This is a lovely way to start your day. Just load up your slow cooker in the evening and leave to cook overnight.

MORNING MILLET

155
calories per
serving

Ingredients

- 250g/9oz millet
- 750ml/3 cups vanilla rice milk
- 3 apples, peeled, cored and chopped
- ¼ tsp each ground cinnamon and nutmeg

TRY COOKING OVERNIGHT

Method

1 Combine all ingredients in the slow cooker and cook on high for 4 hours or on low for 8 hours with the lid tightly shut.

2 Add water if you need to loosen the mixture during cooking.

Family Serving Suggestion (Not 5:2 Followers):
Salad, rolls and barbecue sauce.

CHEFS NOTE
It's best to cook up a large batch of this which the family can share or you can store in the fridge.

Skinny
BREAKFAST
SNACK & LUNCH
RECIPES

MUESLI

124
calories per
serving

Ingredients

- 175g/6oz jumbo oats
- 400g/14oz all bran
- 15g/½oz wheatgerm
- 50g/2oz raisins

- 75g/3oz dried apricots, chopped
- 50g/2oz golden linseeds

Method

Combine all ingredients together and
serve with 120ml skimmed milk.

FRUIT SALAD

138
calories per
serving

Ingredients

- 1 orange
- 1 apple
- 1 banana

- 225g/8oz seedless grapes
- 1 tsp brown sugar

Method

Chop all the fruit and sprinkle with sugar

TUNA & PITTA SALAD

260 calories per serving

Ingredients

- 50g/2oz tinned tuna (in water)
- 2 tsp low fat mayonnaise
- 1 vine ripened tomato, finely chopped
- ½ red onion, finely chopped
- 25g/1oz spinach
- 1 tsp lemon juice
- 2 spring onions chopped
- 1 wholewheat pitta bread

Method

Combine all ingredients together (except pitta) and serve inside the pitta bread.

GRILLED CHICKEN & TOMATO SNACK

SERVES 1

100 calories per serving

Ingredients

- 75g/3oz mini skinless chicken breast
- 100g/3½oz ripe cherry tomatoes, halved
- Low cal cooking spray
- Salt & pepper

Method

1 Spray the chicken and tomatoes with a little low cal oil. Season with plenty of salt and pepper and place under the grill.

2 Leave to cook on a medium heat for 6-10 minutes (or until the chicken is thoroughly cooked). Add some fresh basil or flat leaf parsley to garnish.

CARROT & CELERY SALAD

97
calories per serving

Ingredients

- 2 peeled, grated carrots
- ¼ cucumber, finely chopped
- 1 lemon, juiced
- 2 celery stalks, chopped
- 1 slice of tinned pineapple, chopped
- Pinch of salt

Method

Combine all ingredients well in a bowl.

SUGAR SNAP PEAS WITH SEA SALT

65 calories per serving

Ingredients

- 75g/3oz sugar snap peas
- 1 tsp crushed sea salt
- 1 tsp chopped fresh mint or basil

Method

Place peas in a pan of boiling water for one minute. Drain and mix with salt & herbs.

TUNA, LEMON & CAPERS

100
calories per
serving

Ingredients

- 25g/1oz tinned tuna (in water)
- Squeeze of lemon juice
- 1 tsp capers, finely chopped
- 2 low cal oat cakes

Method

Combine tuna, capers and lemon juice
together and serve on top of oatcakes.

TOMATO, OLIVE & FETA SALAD

113 calories per serving

Ingredients

- 2 tomatoes, sliced
- 1 tsp olive oil
- 25g/1oz low fat feta cheese, crumbled
- 1 tsp fresh basil, chopped
- Splash red wine vinegar
- 1 garlic cloves crushed
- 5 pitted olives
- Salt & pepper

Method

Combine all ingredients well in a bowl.
Season and serve.

SERVES 4

CAULIFLOWER RICE

50
calories per serving

.... *Ingredients* ....

- 1 large head cauliflower

.... *Method* ....

1 Whizz a whole head of cauliflower in the food processor until the pieces are the size of a grain of rice.

2 Microwave in a covered dish for 3-5 minutes and use as substitute for regular rice.

3 Freeze any leftovers into portions.

HOMEMADE SALSA

Ingredients

- 200g/7oz fresh tomatoes, finely chopped
- ½ onion, finely chopped
- 1 green chilli, deseeded & finely chopped
- Small bunch fresh coriander/ cilantro, finely chopped
- Salt & pepper to taste
- Lime juice, to taste
- 1 tbsp water

Method

Combine all ingredients together, balancing the seasoning and lime to your taste. Can be stored for several days in the fridge and used to liven up many meals and snacks.

SERVES 1

STRAWBERRY & BANANA SMOOTHIE

100
calories per serving

Ingredients

- 3 tbsp fat free Greek yoghurt
- ½ banana
- 3 strawberries
- Large handful of ice

Method

Add all the ingredients to the blender
and whizz until smooth.

SERVES 1

MIXED BERRY
SMOOTHIE

100
calories per
serving

Ingredients

- ½ banana
- 50g/2oz mixed soft fruit berries
- 3 tbsp fat free Greek yoghurt
- Large handful of ice

Method

Add all the ingredients to the blender
and whizz until smooth.

KIWI & STRAWBERRY SMOOTHIE

100
calories per
serving

Ingredients

- ½ banana
- ½ kiwi fruit, peeled
- 3 strawberries
- 1 teaspoon Agave nectar
- Large handful of ice

Method

Add all the ingredients to the blender
and whizz until smooth.

CONVERSION CHART: DRY INGREDIENTS

Metric	Imperial
7g	¼ oz
15g	½ oz
20g	¾ oz
25g	1 oz
40g	1½oz
50g	2oz
60g	2½oz
75g	3oz
100g	3½oz
125g	4oz
140g	4½oz
150g	5oz
165g	5½oz
175g	6oz
200g	7oz
225g	8oz
250g	9oz
275g	10oz
300g	11oz
350g	12oz
375g	13oz
400g	14oz

Metric	Imperial
425g	15oz
450g	1lb
500g	1lb 2oz
550g	1¼lb
600g	1lb 5oz
650g	1lb 7oz
675g	1½lb
700g	1lb 9oz
750g	1lb 11oz
800g	1¾lb
900g	2lb
1kg	2¼lb
1.1kg	2½lb
1.25kg	2¾lb
1.35kg	3lb
1.5kg	3lb 6oz
1.8kg	4lb
2kg	4½lb
2.25kg	5lb
2.5kg	5½lb
2.75kg	6lb

CONVERSION CHART: LIQUID MEASURES

Metric	Imperial	US
25ml	1fl oz	
60ml	2fl oz	¼ cup
75ml	2½ fl oz	
100ml	3½fl oz	
120ml	4fl oz	½ cup
150ml	5fl oz	
175ml	6fl oz	
200ml	7fl oz	
250ml	8½ fl oz	1 cup
300ml	10½ fl oz	
360ml	12½ fl oz	
400ml	14fl oz	
450ml	15½ fl oz	
600ml	1 pint	
750ml	1¼ pint	3 cups
1 litre	1½ pints	4 cups

Other
COOKNATION
TITLES

If you enjoyed 'The Skinny 5:2 Diet Slow Cooker Recipe Book' we'd really appreciate your feedback. Reviews help others decide if this is the right book for them.

Thank you.

You may also be interested in other '**Skinny**' titles in the CookNation series. You can find all the following great titles by searching under '**CookNation**'.

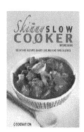

The Skinny Slow Cooker Recipe Book

Delicious Recipes Under 300, 400 And 500 Calories.

Paperback / eBook

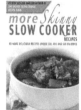

More Skinny Slow Cooker Recipes

75 More Delicious Recipes Under 300, 400 & 500 Calories.

Paperback / eBook

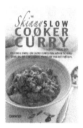

The Skinny Slow Cooker Curry Recipe Book

Low Calorie Curries From Around The World

Paperback / eBook

The Skinny Slow Cooker Soup Recipe Book

Simple, Healthy & Delicious Low Calorie Soup Recipes For Your Slow Cooker. All Under 100, 200 & 300 Calories.

Paperback / eBook

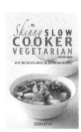

The Skinny Slow Cooker Vegetarian Recipe Book

40 Delicious Recipes Under 200, 300 And 400 Calories.

Paperback / eBook

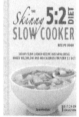

The Skinny 5:2 Slow Cooker Recipe Book

Skinny Slow Cooker Recipe And Menu Ideas Under 100, 200, 300 & 400 Calories For Your 5:2 Diet.

Paperback / eBook

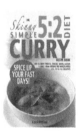

The Skinny 5:2 Curry Recipe Book

Spice Up Your Fast Days With Simple Low Calorie Curries, Snacks, Soups, Salads & Sides Under 200, 300 & 400 Calories

Paperback / eBook

The Skinny Halogen Oven Family Favourites Recipe Book

Healthy, Low Calorie Family Meal-Time Halogen Oven Recipes Under 300, 400 and 500 Calories

Paperback / eBook

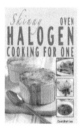

Skinny Halogen Oven Cooking For One

Single Serving, Healthy, Low Calorie Halogen Oven Recipes Under 200, 300 and 400 Calories

Paperback / eBook

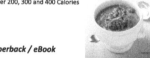

Skinny Winter Warmers Recipe Book

Soups, Stews, Casseroles & One Pot Meals Under 300, 400 & 500 Calories.

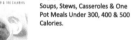

Paperback / eBook

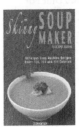

The Skinny Soup Maker Recipe Book
Delicious Low Calorie, Healthy and Simple Soup Recipes Under 100, 200 and 300 Calories. Perfect For Any Diet and Weight Loss Plan.

Paperback / eBook

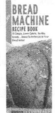

The Skinny Bread Machine Recipe Book
70 Simple, Lower Calorie, Healthy Breads...Baked To Perfection In Your Bread Maker.

Paperback / eBook

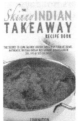

The Skinny Indian Takeaway Recipe Book
Authentic British Indian Restaurant Dishes Under 300, 400 And 500 Calories. The Secret To Low Calorie Indian Takeaway Food At Home

Paperback / eBook

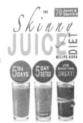

The Skinny Juice Diet Recipe Book
5lbs, 5 Days. The Ultimate Kick-Start Diet and Detox Plan to Lose Weight & Feel Great!

Paperback / eBook

The Skinny 5:2 Diet Recipe Book Collection
All The 5:2 Fast Diet Recipes You'll Ever Need. All Under 100, 200, 300, 400 And 500 Calories

Available only on eBook

eBook

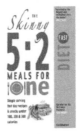

The Skinny 5:2 Fast Diet Meals For One
Single Serving Fast Day Recipes & Snacks Under 100, 200 & 300 Calories

Paperback / eBook

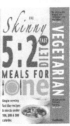

The Skinny 5:2 Fast Diet Vegetarian Meals For One
Single Serving Fast Day Recipes & Snacks Under 100, 200 & 300 Calories

Paperback / eBook

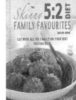

The Skinny 5:2 Fast Diet Family Favourites Recipe Book
Eat With All The Family On Your Diet Fasting Days

Paperback / eBook

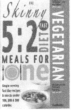

The Skinny 5:2 Fast Diet Family Favorites Recipe Book *U.S.A. EDITION*
Dine With All The Family On Your Diet Fasting Days

Available only on eBook

Paperback / eBook

The Skinny 5:2 Diet Chicken Dishes Recipe Book
Delicious Low Calorie Chicken Dishes Under 300, 400 & 500 Calories

Paperback / eBook

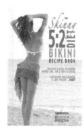

The Skinny 5:2 Bikini Diet Recipe Book

Recipes & Meal Planners Under 100, 200 & 300 Calories. Get Ready For Summer & Lose Weight...FAST!

Paperback / eBook

The Paleo Diet For Beginners Slow Cooker Recipe Book

Gluten Free, Everyday Essential Slow Cooker Paleo Recipes For Beginners

Available only on eBook

eBook

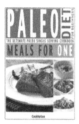

The Paleo Diet For Beginners Meals For One

The Ultimate Paleo Single Serving Cookbook

Paperback / eBook

The Paleo Diet For Beginners Holidays

Thanksgiving, Christmas & New Year Paleo Friendly Recipes

Available only on eBook   *eBook*

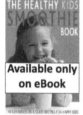

The Healthy Kids Smoothie Book

40 Delicious Goodness In A Glass Recipes for Happy Kids.

eBook

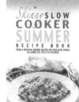

The Skinny Slow Cooker Summer Recipe Book

Fresh & Seasonal Summer Recipes For Your Slow Cooker. All Under 300, 400 And 500 Calories.

Paperback / eBook

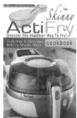
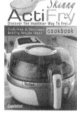

The Skinny ActiFry Cookbook

Guilt-free and Delicious ActiFry Recipe Ideas: Discover The Healthier Way to Fry!

Paperback / eBook

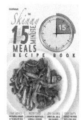

The Skinny 15 Minute Meals Recipe Book

Delicious, Nutritious & Super-Fast Meals in 15 Minutes Or Less. All Under 300, 400 & 500 Calories.

Paperback / eBook

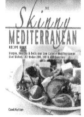

The Skinny Mediterranean Recipe Book

Simple, Healthy & Delicious Low Calorie Mediterranean Diet Dishes. All Under 200, 300 & 400 Calories.

Paperback / eBook

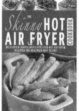

The Skinny Hot Air Fryer Cookbook

Delicious & Simple Meals For Your Hot Air Fryer: Discover The Healthier Way To Fry.

Paperback / eBook

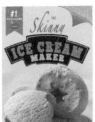

The Skinny Ice Cream Maker

Delicious Lower Fat, Lower Calorie Ice Cream, Frozen Yogurt & Sorbet Recipes For Your Ice Cream Maker

Paperback / eBook

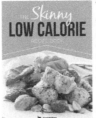

The Skinny Low Calorie Recipe Book

Great Tasting, Simple & Healthy Meals Under 300, 400 & 500 Calories. Perfect For Any Calorie Controlled Diet.

Paperback / eBook

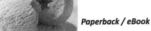

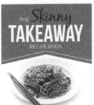

The Skinny Takeaway Recipe Book

Healthier Versions Of Your Fast Food Favourites: Chinese, Indian, Pizza, Burgers, Southern Style Chicken, Mexican & More. All Under 300, 400 & 500 Calories

Paperback / eBook

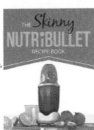

The Skinny Nutribullet Recipe Book

80+ Delicious & Nutritious Healthy Smoothie Recipes. Burn Fat, Lose Weight and Feel Great!

Paperback / eBook

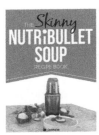

The Skinny Nutribullet Soup Recipe Book

Delicious, Quick & Easy, Single Serving Soups & Pasta Sauces For Your Nutribullet. All Under 100, 200, 300 & 400 Calories.

Paperback / eBook

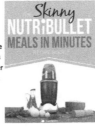

The Skinny Nutribullet Meals In Minutes Recipe Book

Quick & Easy, Single Serving Suppers, Snacks, Sauces, Salad Dressings & More Using Your Nutribullet. All Under 300, 400 & 500 Calories.

Paperback / eBook

Lightning Source UK Ltd.
Milton Keynes UK
UKOW07f0044130115

244382UK00015B/504/P